Discover Chair Yoga

Gentle Fitness for Seniors and Beginners, Seated Exercises for Health and Wellbeing

Jessica Peters

Discover Chair Yoga
Gentle Fitness for Seniors and Beginners, Seated
Exercises for Health and Wellbeing

In association with:
Biz Social Marketing Agency
63 East 11400 South
Suite #230
Sandy, UT 84070
BizSocialMarketing.com

ISBN: 979-8-8692-9618-4

Table of Contents

Disclaimer

The content provided in this book, "Discover Chair Yoga" is intended for informational and educational purposes only. While chair yoga can offer numerous benefits for physical, mental, and emotional well-being, it is essential to consult with a qualified healthcare professional before beginning any new exercise program, especially if you have pre-existing health conditions or concerns.

The information presented in this book is not intended to diagnose, treat, cure, or prevent any disease or medical condition. It should not be used as a substitute for professional medical advice, diagnosis, or treatment. Always seek the advice of your physician or other qualified healthcare provider with any questions you may have regarding your health or a medical condition.

Individual results from practicing chair yoga may vary depending on factors such as age, fitness level, medical history, and adherence to the recommended exercises and guidelines. It is essential to listen to your body and modify or discontinue any exercise that causes discomfort or pain.

By engaging in the practices outlined in this book, you acknowledge and accept full responsibility for your health and well-being. The author and publisher of this book disclaim any liability for any injury, loss, or damage incurred as a result of the use or misuse of the information provided.

Remember, chair yoga is a journey of self-discovery and transformation, and it is essential to approach it with mindfulness, patience, and compassion for yourself. Always prioritize your safety and well-being above all else.

Individual results may vary.

Book Summary Outline

10 Easy Chair Yoga Poses with Instructions

1. Introduction
   - Brief overview of chair yoga and its benefits for weight loss.
   - Explanation of the purpose of the book: to provide low-impact exercises suitable for seniors and beginners.
   - Introduction to the concept of incorporating yoga into daily routine for weight loss.

2. Understanding Chair Yoga
   - Explanation of what chair yoga is and how it differs from traditional yoga.
   - Benefits of chair yoga, particularly its accessibility for those with limited mobility.

- Discussion on the importance of proper posture and alignment during chair yoga practice.

3. The Mind-Body Connection
- Exploration of the mind-body connection in yoga practice.
- Introduction to mindfulness techniques and their role in weight loss.
- Explanation of how chair yoga can promote a positive mindset and support weight loss goals.

4. Harnessing the Power of Breath
- Introduction to pranayama (breath control) techniques.
- Instruction on various breathing exercises suitable for chair yoga practice.
- Explanation of how breath awareness can enhance the effectiveness of chair yoga for weight loss.

5. Warm-Up and Stretching

- Importance of warming up before exercise, especially for seniors and beginners.
- Demonstration of gentle warm-up exercises that can be done in a chair.
- Explanation of the benefits of stretching for weight loss and overall flexibility.

6. Strength-Building Poses
- Introduction to strength-building chair yoga poses.
- Step-by-step instructions for performing poses that target major muscle groups.
- Discussion on how building strength can contribute to weight loss and improved metabolism.

7. Balance and Stability
- Discussion on the importance of balance and stability for overall well-being.
- Demonstration of chair yoga poses that improve balance and stability.

- Tips for modifying poses to accommodate different levels of ability.

8. Flexibility and Range of Motion
- Explanation of the role of flexibility in weight loss and injury prevention.
- Instruction on chair yoga poses that promote flexibility and improve range of motion.
- Discussion on the benefits of maintaining flexibility as we age.

9. Relaxation and Stress Reduction
- Introduction to relaxation techniques in chair yoga.
- Demonstration of poses and breathing exercises for stress reduction.
- Explanation of how managing stress can support weight loss goals.

10. Incorporating Chair Yoga into Daily Life
- Tips for integrating chair yoga into daily routine.

- Suggestions for setting realistic goals and staying motivated.

- Conclusion and encouragement for readers to embrace chair yoga as a tool for weight loss and overall well-being.

11. Appendix: Additional Resources

- List of recommended books, websites, and other resources for further exploration of chair yoga and weight loss.

12. Glossary

- Definitions of key terms and concepts introduced throughout the book.

10 Easy Chair Yoga Poses with Instructions

As we age, it's natural for our bodies to experience changes, and maintaining flexibility, strength, and balance becomes increasingly important. Chair yoga offers a safe and effective way to nurture your body, mind, and spirit, regardless of age or fitness level. In this daily practice, we'll explore a series of easy chair yoga poses that can be seamlessly incorporated into your routine, helping you cultivate greater mobility, relaxation, and inner peace. Whether you're looking to improve flexibility, reduce stress, or simply enhance your quality of life, chair yoga provides a sanctuary for self-care and self-discovery. So, grab a sturdy chair, find a quiet space, and join me on this journey of exploration and transformation. Together, let's embark on a path toward greater health, vitality, and joy through the daily practice of chair yoga.

Spend 10 min a day doing chair yoga. Work up to 30 min a day.

Here are ten easy chair yoga poses along with instructions and pictures:

1. Seated Mountain Pose (Tadasana):

- Sit tall in your chair with your feet flat on the floor.
- Place your hands on your thighs, palms facing down.
- Lengthen your spine, drawing your shoulders back and down.
- Take a few deep breaths, grounding through your sit bones.

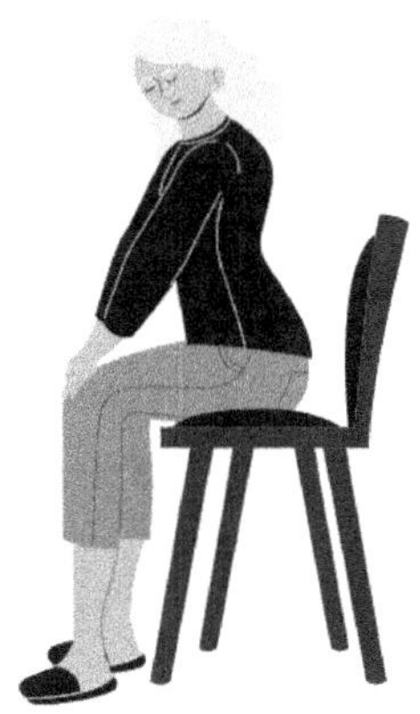

2. Seated Forward Fold (Paschimottanasana):

- Sit tall in your chair with your feet flat on the floor.
- Inhale, lengthen your spine and lift your arms overhead.
- Exhale, hinge at your hips, and fold forward, reaching your hands towards your feet or the floor.
- Keep your back straight and lengthen through your spine.
- Hold for a few breaths, then slowly rise back up on an inhale.

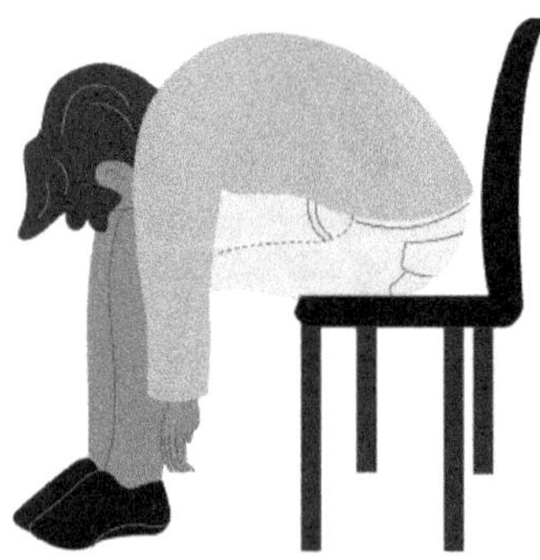

3. Seated Twist (Ardha Matsyendrasana):

- Sit tall in your chair with your feet flat on the floor.
- Inhale, lengthen your spine.
- Exhale, twist to the right, placing your left hand on your right knee and your right hand on the back of the chair.
- Keep your spine tall and twist from your waist.
- Hold for a few breaths, then return to center, and repeat on the other side.

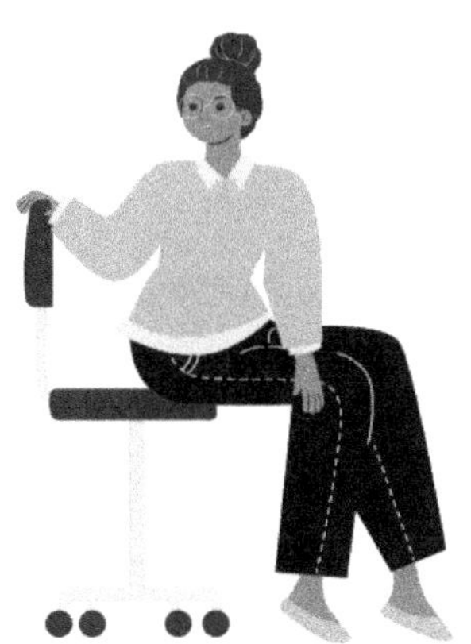

4. Seated Cat-Cow Stretch:

- Sit tall in your chair with your feet flat on the floor.
- Inhale, arch your back and lift your chest towards the ceiling (Cow Pose).
- Exhale, round your spine, and drop your chin towards your chest (Cat Pose).
- Repeat this flowing movement with your breath for several rounds.

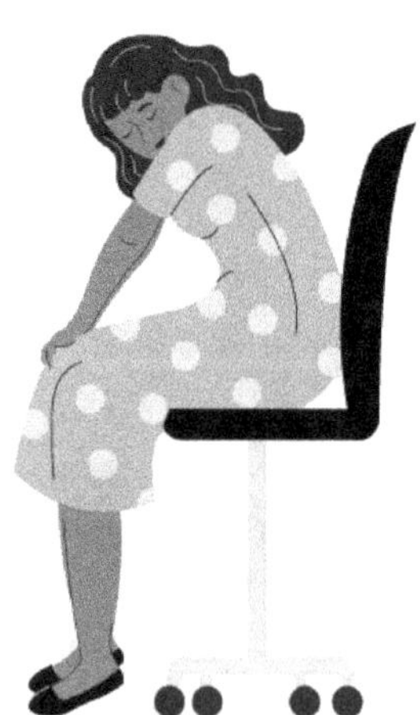

5. Seated Eagle Arms:

- Sit tall in your chair with your feet flat on the floor.
- Inhale, extend your arms out to the sides.
- Exhale, cross your right arm over your left, bending at the elbows.
- Bring your palms together if possible, or simply press the backs of your hands together.
- Hold for a few breaths, then release and repeat on the other side.

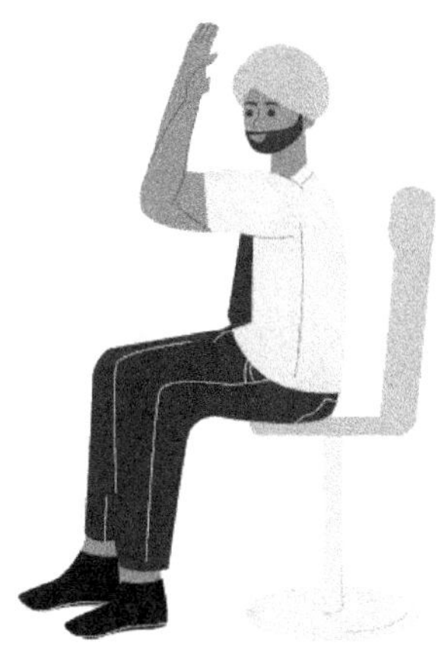

6. Seated Warrior One:

- Sit tall in your chair with your feet flat on the floor.
- Extend your right leg out in front of you, keeping your foot flexed.
- Inhale, reach your arms overhead.
- Exhale, bend your left knee and sink down into a lunge position.
- Keep your spine tall and engage your core.
- Hold for a few breaths, then switch sides.

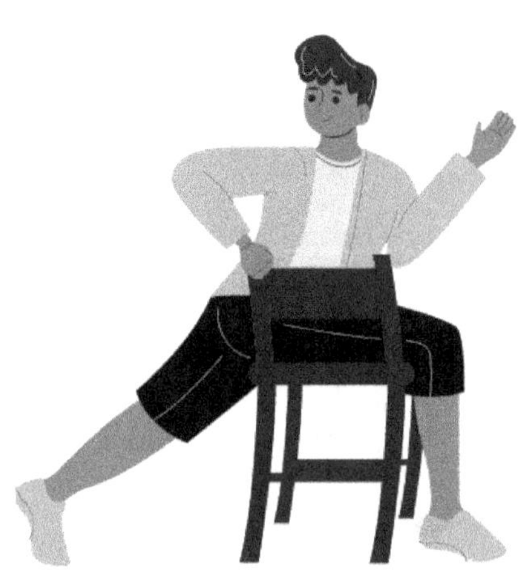

7. Seated Warrior Two:

- Sit tall in your chair with your feet flat on the floor.
- Extend your right leg out in front of you, keeping your foot flexed.
- Turn your torso to the right and extend your arms out to the sides, parallel to the floor.
- Bend your left knee and sink down into a lunge position.
- Keep your gaze over your right fingertips and your spine tall.
- Hold for a few breaths, then switch sides.

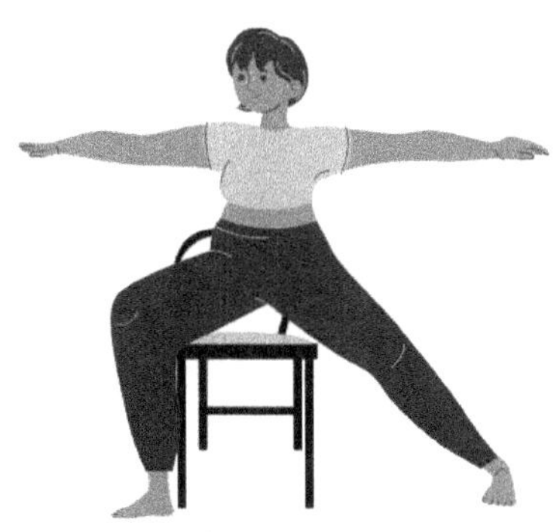

8. Seated Pigeon Pose:

- Sit tall in your chair with your feet flat on the floor.
- Cross your right ankle over your left knee, flexing your right foot.
- Inhale, lengthen your spine.
- Exhale, hinge forward at your hips, keeping your back straight.
- Hold for a few breaths, then switch sides.

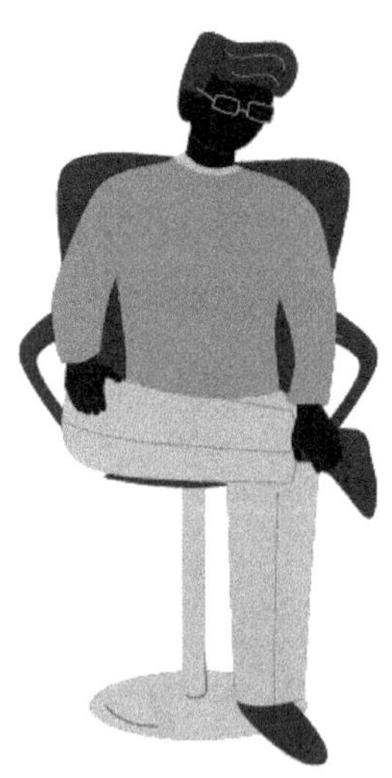

9. Seated Shoulder Stretch:

- Sit tall in your chair with your feet flat on the floor.
- Reach your right arm across your chest, placing your left hand on your right elbow.
- Gently press your right arm towards your chest until you feel a stretch in your shoulder.
- Hold for a few breaths, then switch sides.

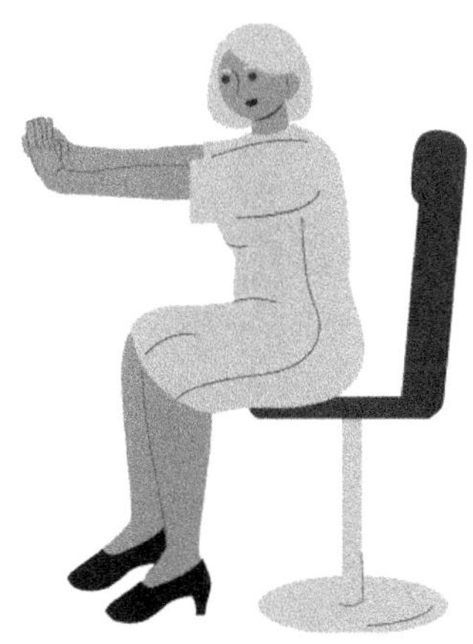

10. Seated Neck Stretch:

- Sit tall in your chair with your feet flat on the floor.
- Drop your right ear towards your right shoulder, stretching the left side of your neck.
- Gently place your right hand on the top of your head to deepen the stretch.
- Hold for a few breaths, then switch sides.

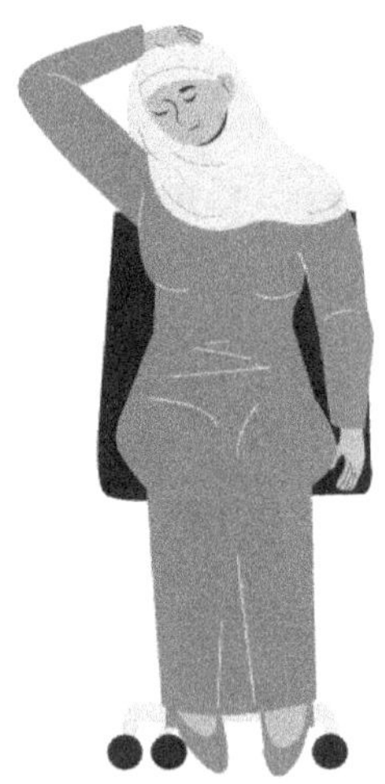

These chair yoga poses are gentle and accessible for beginners and can be practiced virtually anywhere, making them ideal for incorporating into your daily routine for improved flexibility, relaxation, and overall well-being.

Introduction

Welcome to "Discover Chair Yoga" In this book, we embark on a journey that blends the ancient wisdom of yoga with modern fitness principles to achieve tangible results in weight loss, all from the comfort of a chair.

As a seasoned fitness authority deeply rooted in the daily practice of yoga, I've witnessed firsthand the transformative power of this ancient discipline. Yoga is not merely a series of physical postures; it is a holistic approach to wellness that nurtures the body, mind, and spirit. And chair yoga, with its gentle yet effective movements, opens the door to this transformative experience for individuals of all ages and fitness levels, especially seniors and beginners.

Our focus here is on harnessing the innate potential of chair yoga to aid in weight loss. But let me be clear: this is not a quick-fix solution promising overnight results. Instead, it's a sustainable approach that advocates for consistency and mindful practice. By dedicating just 10 minutes a day to these low-impact exercises, you can embark on a journey toward a healthier, more vibrant you.

Throughout this book, we'll delve into the fundamentals of chair yoga, exploring its unique benefits and the profound connection between body and mind. We'll learn how simple breathing techniques can enhance our practice and support our weight loss goals. We'll discover a curated selection of poses designed to strengthen muscles, improve balance, and increase flexibility – essential elements in any successful weight loss journey.

But beyond the physical aspects, we'll also explore the importance of relaxation and stress reduction in achieving sustainable weight loss. Yoga teaches us to cultivate awareness and presence, empowering us to make conscious choices that align with our well-being.

So, whether you're a seasoned yogi looking for a new approach or a complete novice eager to explore the transformative potential of yoga, this book is for you. Together, let's embark on this journey toward a healthier, happier self – one mindful breath and gentle movement at a time.

Chapter One:
Understanding Chair Yoga

As we embark on our journey to explore chair yoga, it's essential to first grasp the fundamental principles that underpin this ancient practice. Chair yoga is not merely a modification of traditional yoga; it is a unique discipline tailored to meet the needs of individuals with varying levels of mobility and fitness. In this chapter, we will delve into the essence of chair yoga, shedding light on its benefits and offering insights into its transformative potential.

At its core, chair yoga is about accessibility and inclusivity. It recognizes that yoga is for every body, regardless of age, ability, or physical limitations. By utilizing a chair as a prop, we can adapt traditional yoga poses to accommodate individuals who may find it challenging to practice on the mat. Whether you're a senior looking to maintain flexibility, a beginner easing into fitness, or someone recovering from injury, chair yoga offers a safe and supportive environment for exploration and growth.

One of the key benefits of chair yoga lies in its emphasis on proper alignment and posture. With the support of a chair, practitioners can focus on aligning their bodies correctly, reducing the risk of strain or injury. This attention to alignment enhances the effectiveness of the poses and cultivates a deeper awareness of the body-mind connection – a cornerstone of yoga philosophy.

Furthermore, chair yoga serves as a gateway to mindfulness and self-awareness. As we move through the poses with intention and breath awareness, we are invited to be fully present in the moment, letting go of distractions and cultivating a sense of inner peace. This mindfulness practice extends beyond the mat, empowering us to navigate life's challenges with grace and resilience.

In understanding chair yoga, it's essential to recognize its versatility and adaptability. Whether you're practicing in the comfort of your living room or participating in a group class at a community center, chair yoga can be tailored to suit your individual needs and preferences. With a bit of creativity and an open mind, you can incorporate chair yoga into your daily routine, reaping its myriad benefits wherever you go.

As we journey deeper into the world of chair yoga, remember that it's not about perfection but progress. Embrace the process, listen to your body, and honor your unique journey. Together, let's unlock the transformative power of chair yoga and embark on a path to greater health, vitality, and well-being.

Chapter Two:
The Essence of Chair Yoga

In the vast landscape of yoga, chair yoga stands out as a beacon of accessibility and inclusivity, offering a gateway for individuals of all ages and abilities to embark on a journey of self-discovery and transformation. In this chapter, we will delve into the essence of chair yoga – its origins, its philosophy, and its unique approach to wellness.

At its core, chair yoga embodies the principle of adaptation – the art of modifying traditional yoga poses to suit the needs of diverse practitioners. By incorporating a chair as a prop, we can create a supportive environment that empowers individuals with limited mobility or physical challenges to experience the benefits of yoga firsthand. Whether you are recovering from injury, managing chronic pain, or simply seeking a gentle introduction to fitness, chair yoga welcomes you with open arms.

But beyond its practical applications, chair yoga embodies a deeper philosophy rooted in the ancient wisdom of yoga. At its heart, yoga is a holistic practice that seeks to unite body, mind, and spirit, fostering a sense of wholeness and integration. Chair yoga honors this tradition, offering a holistic approach to wellness that transcends the physical world.

One of the hallmarks of chair yoga is its emphasis on mindfulness – the practice of cultivating awareness and presence in the moment. As we move through the poses with intention and breath awareness, we are invited to quiet the chatter of the mind and tune into the wisdom of the body. This mindfulness practice enhances the effectiveness of the poses and fosters a deeper sense of connection with ourselves and the world around us.

Furthermore, chair yoga serves as a vehicle for self-expression and creativity, inviting practitioners to explore movement and breath in a way that feels authentic and empowering. Whether you're flowing through a sequence of gentle stretches or finding stillness in a seated meditation, chair yoga offers a canvas for self-discovery and exploration.

In embracing the essence of chair yoga, we honor the diversity of human experience and celebrate the inherent beauty of every individual. Regardless of age, ability, or background, chair yoga invites us to come as we are, embracing our strengths and limitations with grace and compassion.

As we journey deeper into the world of chair yoga, may we cultivate an attitude of openness and curiosity, allowing ourselves to be guided by the wisdom of our bodies and the teachings of this ancient practice. Together, let us embark on a path of self-discovery and transformation, one breath and one pose at a time.

Chapter Three:
The Mind-Body Connection

In the world of fitness and yoga, the concept of the mind-body connection is more than just a buzzword – it's a fundamental principle that guides our practice and informs our understanding of holistic wellness. In this chapter, we'll delve into the profound relationship between the mind and body, exploring how chair yoga serves as a powerful tool for nurturing this connection and fostering inner harmony.

At its essence, the mind-body connection is about recognizing the interplay between our thoughts, emotions, and physical sensations. In the fast-paced world we inhabit, it's all too easy to become disconnected from our bodies, operating on autopilot as we rush from one task to the next. However, through the practice of chair yoga, we have the opportunity to rekindle this connection, tuning in to the subtle cues and signals that our bodies send us.

One of the primary ways in which chair yoga facilitates this connection is through breath awareness. As we move through the poses, we are encouraged to synchronize our breath with our movements, fostering a sense of flow and rhythm. This conscious breathing not only oxygenates our muscles but also calms the mind, helping us to cultivate a state of relaxation and presence.

Moreover, chair yoga invites us to cultivate mindfulness – the practice of being fully present in the moment, without judgment or attachment. By directing our attention inward, we can observe our thoughts and sensations with curiosity and compassion, gaining insight into the workings of our minds. This mindfulness practice is not limited to the confines of the yoga mat; rather, it permeates every aspect of our lives, empowering us to approach challenges with clarity and equanimity.

Through the mind-body connection cultivated in chair yoga, we begin to recognize the innate wisdom of our bodies – a wisdom that is often overshadowed by the noise of daily life. By honoring our bodies and listening to their signals, we can learn to move with greater ease and grace, both on and off the mat. In doing so, we awaken to a deeper sense of self-awareness and self-compassion, laying the foundation for profound transformation and growth.

As we continue our journey of exploration, let us remember the inherent interconnectedness of mind and body – a symbiotic relationship that holds the key to our well-being. Through the practice of chair yoga, may we deepen our understanding of this connection and embrace the transformative power it holds.

Chapter Four: Harnessing the Power of Breath

Breath is a physiological function; it is a powerful tool for cultivating awareness, promoting relaxation, and fostering transformation. In this chapter, we will explore the profound role that breath plays in our daily practice, and how harnessing its power can deepen our connection to body, mind, and spirit.

Breath is the bridge that links the external world with our inner landscape, serving as a constant reminder of our innate vitality and presence. In chair yoga, we have the opportunity to tap into this vital force, using it as a guide to navigate our practice with grace and intention. By cultivating a conscious awareness of our breath, we can synchronize our movements, quiet the fluctuations of the mind, and cultivate a sense of inner calm.

One of the primary ways in which breath enhances our chair yoga practice is through its ability to regulate the nervous system. By engaging in slow, deep breathing techniques, such as diaphragmatic breathing or ujjayi breath, we can activate the parasympathetic nervous system – the body's natural relaxation response. This shift from "fight or flight" mode to "rest and digest" mode promotes a sense of calm and tranquility and supports our overall health and well-being.

Moreover, breath serves as a powerful tool for cultivating mindfulness – the practice of being fully present in the moment, without judgment or attachment. As we tune into the rhythm of our breath, we become more attuned to the sensations of our bodies, the thoughts in our minds, and the emotions in our hearts. This mindfulness practice enhances the effectiveness of our chair yoga poses and deepens our connection to ourselves and the world around us.

In chair yoga, breath is our constant companion – a source of strength, stability, and solace amidst the ebb and flow of life. Whether we're flowing through a sequence of dynamic movements or finding stillness in a seated meditation, breath remains our steadfast anchor, guiding us back to the present moment again and again.

As we continue our journey of exploration, let us remember the transformative power of breath – a force that has the potential to awaken us to the fullness of our being. Through the practice of chair yoga, may we cultivate a deeper awareness of our breath and harness its power to nourish our bodies, calm our minds, and uplift our spirits.

Chapter Five:
Invigorating Warm-Up and Blissful Stretching

Before delving into the depths of chair yoga practice, it's essential to lay a solid foundation through invigorating warm-up exercises and blissful stretching routines. In this chapter, we'll explore the importance of preparing the body and mind for movement, and we'll discover a selection of gentle yet effective warm-up and stretching techniques to ignite our practice.

Warm-up exercises serve as the gateway to a successful chair yoga session, priming the body for movement and enhancing circulation. By engaging in dynamic movements that target major muscle groups, we awaken dormant energy and prepare the body for deeper exploration. These exercises prevent injury and cultivate a sense of vitality and presence, setting the stage for a fulfilling yoga experience.

In chair yoga, we have the unique opportunity to explore a wide range of warm-up exercises that can be performed from the comfort of our seats. From gentle neck rolls and shoulder shrugs to seated twists and side stretches, these movements help lubricate the joints, improve the range of motion, and release tension held in the body. As we flow through these invigorating warm-up exercises, we invite a sense of openness and receptivity, allowing the energy to flow freely throughout our entire being.

Following our warm-up, we transition seamlessly into the world of stretching – a practice that nourishes the body, soothes the mind, and promotes flexibility. Stretching is not merely about lengthening muscles; it's about honoring the body's innate wisdom and tuning into the subtle sensations that arise with each movement. In chair yoga, we have the opportunity to explore a variety of stretching techniques that cater to our individual needs and preferences.

From seated forward folds and gentle backbends to hamstring stretches and hip openers, these stretching routines offer a sanctuary for self-care and rejuvenation. As we sink deeper into each stretch, we breathe life into stiff joints, release stored tension, and cultivate a profound sense of relaxation. With each exhale, we surrender to the present moment, allowing our bodies to soften and our minds to quieten.

In embracing the practice of warm-up and stretching in chair yoga, we honor the inherent wisdom of the body and celebrate the journey of self-discovery and self-care. As we move through these invigorating warm-up exercises and blissful stretching routines, may we cultivate an attitude of curiosity and compassion, embracing the fullness of our experience with grace and gratitude.

Together, let us embark on a journey of exploration and transformation, igniting our practice with the radiant warmth of intention and the blissful expansiveness of stretching.

Chapter Six:
Empowering Strength-Building Poses

In the world of chair yoga, the quest for strength is not limited by physical limitations or age; it is a journey of empowerment that transcends boundaries and celebrates the resilience of the human spirit. In this chapter, we will explore a curated selection of strength-building poses designed to ignite the fire within, sculpt lean muscles, and cultivate a sense of vitality and resilience.

Strength-building poses in chair yoga offer a unique opportunity to harness the power of resistance and engage in dynamic movements that challenge our bodies and minds. These poses are not about brute force or competition; they are about tapping into our inner reservoir of strength and embracing the journey of self-discovery and growth.

At the heart of strength-building poses lies the principle of stability – the ability to find balance and support within ourselves, even in the face of adversity. Whether we're flowing through dynamic sequences or holding steady in static poses, stability serves as our steadfast anchor, grounding us in the present moment and fostering a sense of inner strength and resilience.

One of the key benefits of strength-building poses in chair yoga is their ability to target major muscle groups while minimizing strain on the joints. From seated squats and leg lifts to arm circles and bicep curls, these poses offer a full-body workout that strengthens muscles, improves posture, and enhances overall functionality. As we move through these empowering poses, we cultivate a deeper awareness of our bodies and develop a greater appreciation for their inherent strength and resilience.

Moreover, strength-building poses in chair yoga offers a sanctuary for self-exploration and self-expression, inviting us to step into our power and embrace the fullness of our potential. As we engage in these empowering poses, we cultivate a sense of confidence and empowerment that extends far beyond the confines of the yoga mat.

In embracing the practice of strength-building poses in chair yoga, we honor the strength and resilience that resides within each of us. As we flow through these empowering poses, may we embrace the journey of self-discovery and growth with courage and compassion, trusting in our ability to rise above challenges and thrive in the face of adversity.

Together, let us unleash the power of strength-building poses in chair yoga, igniting the fire within and embracing the transformative journey ahead.

Chapter Seven: Cultivating Balance and Stability

In the dynamic world of chair yoga, balance, and stability are not merely physical attributes; they are essential pillars of well-being that support us on our journey of self-discovery and transformation. In this chapter, we will explore a series of gentle yet effective chair yoga poses designed to cultivate balance, enhance stability, and foster a sense of groundedness and presence.

Balance and stability are foundational elements of a strong and resilient body, offering support and protection against injury and falls. In chair yoga, we have the opportunity to explore a variety of poses that challenge our equilibrium and invite us to find steadiness amidst movement. From seated tree pose and eagle arms to modified warrior III and chair squats, these poses offer a sanctuary for self-exploration and growth.

At the heart of balance and stability lies the principle of alignment – the art of finding harmony and integration within ourselves and the world around us. As we move through these balancing poses with grace and intention, we cultivate a deeper awareness of our bodies and develop a greater appreciation for their innate wisdom and resilience. With each breath, we ground ourselves in the present moment, allowing the energy to flow freely throughout our entire being.

One of the key benefits of balance and stability poses in chair yoga is their ability to strengthen the muscles that support our joints, improving overall functionality and mobility. As we engage in these empowering poses, we develop a greater sense of confidence and self-assurance that extends far beyond the confines of the yoga mat.

Moreover, balance and stability poses in chair yoga offer a sanctuary for self-discovery and self-expression, inviting us to explore the edges of our comfort zone and embrace the fullness of our potential. As we navigate the ebb and flow of these dynamic poses, we cultivate a sense of resilience and adaptability that serves us well in all areas of our lives.

In embracing the practice of balance and stability poses in chair yoga, we honor the interconnectedness of body, mind, and spirit, and celebrate the journey of self-discovery and growth. As we flow through these empowering poses, may we embrace the beauty of impermanence and find peace in the ever-changing dance of life.

Together, let us cultivate balance and stability in chair yoga, anchoring ourselves in the present moment and embracing the transformative journey ahead.

Chapter Eight:
Embracing Flexibility and Range of Motion

In the world of chair yoga, flexibility is not merely about bending the body into pretzel-like shapes; it is about cultivating a sense of openness and freedom that extends far beyond the physical realm. In this chapter, we will explore a series of gentle yet profound chair yoga poses designed to enhance flexibility, improve range of motion, and foster a deeper connection to body, mind, and spirit.

Flexibility is a cornerstone of physical health and well-being, offering a sanctuary for self-exploration and growth. In chair yoga, we have the opportunity to explore a variety of poses that gently stretch and lengthen the muscles, releasing tension and promoting relaxation. From seated forward folds and gentle twists to modified pigeon pose and hamstring stretches, these poses offer a refuge for self-care and rejuvenation.

At the heart of flexibility lies the principle of surrender – the art of letting go and embracing the present moment with open arms. As we move through these gentle stretches with grace and ease, we cultivate a deeper awareness of our bodies and develop a greater appreciation for their innate wisdom and resilience. With each breath, we surrender to the flow of life, allowing the energy to flow freely throughout our entire being.

One of the key benefits of flexibility poses in chair yoga is their ability to improve joint mobility and function, reducing the risk of injury and enhancing overall quality of life. As we engage in these empowering poses, we cultivate a sense of spaciousness and freedom that extends far beyond the confines of the yoga mat.

Moreover, flexibility poses in chair yoga offer a sanctuary for self-discovery and self-expression, inviting us to explore the edges of our comfort zone and embrace the fullness of our potential. As we navigate the ebb and flow of these dynamic poses, we cultivate a sense of resilience and adaptability that serves us well in all areas of our lives.

In embracing the practice of flexibility poses in chair yoga, we honor the interconnectedness of body, mind, and spirit, and celebrate the journey of self-discovery and growth. As we flow through these empowering poses, may we embrace the beauty of impermanence and find peace in the ever-changing dance of life.

Together, let us cultivate flexibility and range of motion in chair yoga, anchoring ourselves in the present moment and embracing the transformative journey ahead.

Chapter Nine:
Nurturing Relaxation and Stress Reduction

In the fast-paced world we inhabit, relaxation and stress reduction have become essential pillars of well-being, offering a sanctuary for self-care and rejuvenation amidst the chaos of daily life. In this chapter, we will explore a series of gentle yet profound chair yoga poses and techniques designed to nurture relaxation, promote stress reduction, and cultivate a deeper sense of peace and tranquility.

Relaxation is not merely the absence of tension; it is a state of being characterized by ease, comfort, and surrender. In chair yoga, we have the opportunity to explore a variety of relaxation techniques that gently soothe the nervous system and invite us to sink deeper into a state of profound relaxation. From guided meditation and body scans to progressive muscle relaxation and breath awareness, these techniques offer a refuge for self-exploration and self-discovery.

At the heart of relaxation lies the principle of surrender – the art of letting go and embracing the present moment with open arms. As we engage in these gentle practices with grace and ease, we cultivate a deeper awareness of our bodies and develop a greater appreciation for their innate wisdom and resilience. With each breath, we surrender to the flow of life, allowing the energy to flow freely throughout our entire being.

One of the key benefits of relaxation techniques in chair yoga is their ability to soothe the nervous system, reduce stress hormones, and promote a sense of inner calm and peace. As we engage in these empowering practices, we cultivate a sense of spaciousness and freedom that extends far beyond the confines of the yoga mat.

Moreover, relaxation techniques in chair yoga offer a sanctuary for self-discovery and self-expression, inviting us to explore the depths of our inner landscape and embrace the fullness of our potential. As we navigate the ebb and flow of these dynamic practices, we cultivate a sense of resilience and adaptability that serves us well in all areas of our lives.

In embracing the practice of relaxation and stress reduction in chair yoga, we honor the interconnectedness of body, mind, and spirit, and celebrate the journey of self-discovery and growth. As we flow through these empowering practices, may we embrace the beauty of impermanence and find peace in the ever-changing dance of life.

Together, let us nurture relaxation and stress reduction in chair yoga, anchoring ourselves in the present moment and embracing the transformative journey ahead.

Chapter Ten:
Integrating Chair Yoga into Daily Life

As we near the culmination of our journey through chair yoga, it's essential to reflect on how we can integrate the wisdom and practices we've cultivated into our daily lives. In this chapter, we'll explore practical strategies for incorporating chair yoga into our routines, setting realistic goals, and staying motivated on our path to wellness and transformation.

Chair yoga offers a gateway to holistic well-being that extends far beyond the confines of the yoga mat. By embracing its principles and practices, we can enhance our physical health, nurture our emotional well-being, and cultivate a deeper sense of connection to ourselves and the world around us. But to truly reap the benefits of chair yoga, we must find ways to weave its teachings into the fabric of our daily lives.

One of the first steps in integrating chair yoga into our daily routine is to set realistic goals that align with our intentions and aspirations. Whether it's committing to a daily 10-minute practice or attending a weekly chair yoga class, setting achievable goals allows us to stay focused and motivated on our path to wellness. By breaking our goals down into manageable steps and celebrating our progress along the way, we can build momentum and cultivate a sense of accomplishment that fuels our journey.

Moreover, finding moments of mindfulness and presence in our daily lives can serve as a powerful complement to our formal chair yoga practice. Whether it's taking a few deep breaths before a stressful meeting, practicing gratitude before bed, or simply savoring a moment of stillness with a cup of tea, these small moments of mindfulness can help us stay grounded and centered amidst the busyness of life.

Another key aspect of integrating chair yoga into daily life is finding support and accountability from like-minded individuals. Whether it's joining a chair yoga community online, participating in a local yoga class, or simply sharing our experiences with friends and loved ones, connecting with others on a similar journey can provide encouragement, inspiration, and camaraderie along the way.

In embracing the practice of chair yoga as a way of life, we honor the interconnectedness of body, mind, and spirit, and celebrate the journey of self-discovery and growth. As we navigate the ups and downs of daily life, may we find solace and strength in the teachings of chair yoga, anchoring ourselves in the present moment and embracing the transformative journey ahead.

Together, let us integrate chair yoga into our daily lives, nourishing our bodies, minds, and spirits with each breath and each movement, and embracing the radiant beauty of the present moment.

Appendix: Additional Resources

As you continue your journey of exploration and growth in chair yoga, you may find it helpful to dive deeper into the wealth of resources available. Below are some recommended books and online resources to further support your practice and enhance your understanding of chair yoga and its transformative potential.

Books and accessories:

1. "Chair Yoga: Sit, Stretch, and Strengthen Your Way to a Happier, Healthier You" by Kristin McGee

- This comprehensive guide offers a variety of chair yoga routines designed to improve flexibility, build strength, and reduce stress. With clear instructions and illustrations, it's perfect for beginners and seasoned practitioners alike.

2. "Yoga XXL: A Journey to Health for Bigger People" by Ingrid Kollak

- In this accessible guide, Ingrid Kollak shares a series of gentle chair yoga poses specifically tailored for bigger people. With an emphasis on safety and effectiveness, this book is a valuable resource for XXL adults looking to maintain flexibility and mobility.

3. "28 Days of Chair Yoga For Seniors Build Strength, Boost Flexibility, and Increase Balance in Just 10 Minutes a Day" by Ottie Oz

- Ottie Oz provides easy-to-follow instructions for 28 days of chair yoga suitable for seniors and beginners. With modifications and variations included, this book offers a gentle introduction to the practice of chair yoga.

4. "Yoga Auxiliary Chair Foldable Backless Yoga Chair with Purple Yoga Resistance Band for Abs & Core, Flexibility and Strength Training and Back Pain Relieving"

- Backless Yoga Chair - Substandard yoga asanas are prone to injury. The Backless Yoga Chair is designed for yoga practice and helps practitioners to better master the asanas, helping to stretch and correct posture while improving blood circulation, strengthening core muscles, and soothing back and neck pain

Online Resources

1. Yoga with Adriene (YouTube Channel)

   - Adriene Mishler offers a variety of chair yoga videos on her popular YouTube channel. With her warm and encouraging teaching style, she guides viewers through gentle chair yoga sequences suitable for all levels.

2. DoYogaWithMe.com

   - This website offers a collection of chair yoga classes led by experienced instructors. From gentle stretches to strength-building poses, there's something for everyone looking to explore chair yoga from the comfort of their home.

3. The Yoga Alliance

- The Yoga Alliance website provides a directory of registered yoga teachers and studios offering chair yoga classes in your area. Whether you're looking for in-person or online classes, you can use this resource to find a qualified instructor near you.

Remember, the journey of chair yoga is unique to each individual, and there's no one-size-fits-all approach. Explore these resources with an open mind and heart, and trust in your intuition to guide you toward the practices and teachings that resonate most deeply with you.

Happy exploring, and may your chair yoga journey be filled with joy, vitality, and transformation.

Glossary

As you dive deeper into the practice of chair yoga, you may encounter terms and concepts that are unfamiliar or require clarification. This glossary provides definitions for key terms used throughout the book, helping you navigate your journey with greater ease and understanding.

1. Chair Yoga: A form of yoga that adapts traditional yoga poses to be performed while seated or using a chair for support. Chair yoga is suitable for individuals of all ages and abilities, including seniors and those with limited mobility.

2. Breath Awareness: The practice of paying attention to the breath, and observing its rhythm and sensations as a way to cultivate mindfulness and presence during yoga practice.

3. Pranayama: The practice of breath control in yoga, consisting of various breathing techniques that aim to regulate the flow of prana (life force energy) in the body and calm the mind.

4. Mindfulness: The practice of being fully present in the moment, without judgment or attachment, and cultivating awareness of one's thoughts, emotions, and sensations.

5. Warm-Up: A series of gentle movements and stretches performed at the beginning of a yoga practice to prepare the body for more intense physical activity and reduce the risk of injury.

6. Stretching: The practice of elongating the muscles and soft tissues of the body to improve flexibility, increase range of motion, and reduce stiffness.

7. Strength-Building Poses: Yoga poses that target specific muscle groups to build strength and stability in the body, improving posture and enhancing overall physical function.

8. Balance: The ability to maintain equilibrium and stability in the body, both physically and mentally, often achieved through yoga poses that challenge proprioception and coordination.

9. Stability: The state of being firm, steady, and grounded in the body, often achieved through yoga poses that engage the core muscles and promote alignment.

10. Flexibility: The ability of the muscles and joints to move freely through their full range of motion, often achieved through stretching and yoga poses that lengthen the muscles and increase mobility.

11. Relaxation: The state of physical and mental ease and calmness, often achieved through relaxation techniques such as deep breathing, guided meditation, and progressive muscle relaxation.

12. Stress Reduction: The practice of minimizing or managing stress through various techniques, including yoga, meditation, mindfulness, and relaxation.

13. Integration: The process of incorporating yoga practices and teachings into daily life, cultivating a holistic approach to health and well-being that extends beyond the yoga mat.

14. Mind-Body Connection: The recognition of the interdependence and interaction between the mind and body, emphasizing the importance of nurturing both physical and mental health through yoga and mindfulness practices.

Refer to this glossary whenever you encounter unfamiliar terms or concepts, and use it as a reference to deepen your understanding of chair yoga and its transformative potential.

Acknowledgments

I would like to express my deepest gratitude to everyone who has contributed to the creation of this book, "Discover Chair Yoga"

First and foremost, I extend my heartfelt appreciation to the dedicated team at Biz Social Marketing, whose expertise and support have been invaluable throughout every stage of the publishing process. Your commitment to excellence and passion for promoting wellness through literature has truly made this project possible.

I am immensely grateful to my yoga mentors and teachers, whose wisdom, guidance, and inspiration have shaped my understanding of chair yoga and its transformative potential. Your dedication to the practice and your unwavering commitment to sharing its benefits with others has been a constant source of motivation and inspiration. Rebecca Walton, I miss the Zoom Yoga we used to do in 2020 and 2021.

I extend my sincere thanks to the individuals who graciously shared their stories, insights, and experiences with chair yoga, enriching the content of this book and providing real-world examples of its impact on health and wellbeing. Your openness and willingness to contribute have added depth and authenticity to these pages.

Last but not least, I extend my deepest appreciation to the readers of this book.

It is my hope that the practices and teachings shared within these pages will serve as a source of inspiration, empowerment, and transformation on your journey to greater health, vitality, and well-being.

With gratitude,

–Jessica Peters